HIGH BLOOD

Explains the working of the circulatory system, points
out the threat to its efficient function posed by high-
cholesterol foods, and lays down guidelines for over-
coming high blood pressure.

HIGH BLOOD PRESSURE

Prepared and produced by the Editorial Committee of Science of Life Books

Revised and Extended by
Leonard Mervyn B.Sc., Ph.D., F.R.S.C.

SCIENCE OF LIFE BOOKS
4-12 Tattersalls Lane, Melbourne, Victoria 3000

Eleventh Edition, revised
and reset, 1982
Second Impression 1983

© SCIENCE OF LIFE BOOKS 1982

*Registered at the G.P.O. Sydney
for transmission through the post
as a book*

*This book is sold subject to the condition that it shall not, by way of
trade or otherwise, be lent, re-sold, hired out, or otherwise circulated
without the publisher's prior consent in any form of binding or cover
other than that in which it is published and without a similar condition
including this condition being imposed on the subsequent purchaser.*

British Library Cataloguing in Publication Data

High blood pressure.—11th ed.
 1. Hypertension   2. Naturopathy
616.'32065   RA645.49

ISBN 0-909911-96-7

National Library of Australia card number
and ISBN 0 909911 96 7

Typeset by Harper Phototypesetters, Northampton.
Printed and bound in Great Britain by
Richard Clay (The Chaucer Press) Limited,
Bungay, Suffolk.

Contents

Introduction

For many people high blood pressure has become more than just a chronic complaint, it is a way of life; a way of life dependent upon drug medication and regular visits to the doctor for repeat prescriptions and check-ups.

Statistics issued by the National Heart Foundation of Australia reveal that some 1,200,000 Australians (15 per cent of all adults in Australia) have raised blood pressure. Unfortunately, one third of these people are unaware of their condition and all too often high blood pressure remains undetected until it has reached dangerously high levels.

High blood pressure contributes considerably to cardiovascular disease and heart trouble. Approximately 40 per cent of all deaths in Australia are due to circulatory disorders. Similar figures exist in other modern Western countries such as U.S.A., the United Kingdom, New Zealand and Northern Europe.

High blood pressure or hypertension and arterio-sclerosis (hardened arteries) are two basic conditions which underlie many forms of cardiovascular disease.

Moreover, it is not unusual for high blood pressure to cause kidney trouble.

This picture is an unpleasant one and one which indeed gives us cause for concern. Medical treatment, for the most part, offers no cure, only relief from hypotensive drugs. Some of these drugs not only lower the blood pressure but also cause undesirable side effects some of which can be quite serious. One of the more common of these side effects is tiredness and extreme lack of energy. These unfortunate people often seek vitamins and other supplements to overcome this tiredness when actually the only satisfactory treatment is to discontinue taking the drugs which caused it. Many people are faced with a dilemma: which is the worst of two evils, the disease or the cure? They are afraid not to use the prescribed drugs and, at the same time, they want to avoid the side effects that accompany their use. What is the answer? What hope do these sufferers have? The information contained in this book provides an answer for many and in most cases will help to provide a solution to their problem, a solution which is not based on treating the disease, or on using artificial methods to suppress the blood pressure but on studying the nature of the complaint and removing the cause. If the cause can be removed, then the patient's own natural recuperative powers can take over and restore health so that drugs become unnecessary and there are no side effects.

Fifty years ago, high blood pressure was relatively uncommon. What has happened during the last half century that could have caused such an increase in this disease? Clearly high blood pressure must be linked to modern lifestyles and diet. It has been demonstrated that rich foods, too much fat, too much sugar and too much common salt in our diet are all important factors contributing to high blood pressure.

Needless to say, overweight and high blood pressure go hand in hand. One of the first considerations in the treatment of high blood pressure should be to reduce body weight to normal levels. One of the major health problems in Western countries is overweight. All too often in affluent areas, people are overfed but undernourished. In Australia for example, statistics show that 25 per cent of energy (calories) available comes from alcohol and white sugar.

Smoking can also play an important role in contributing to high blood pressure. Cigarettes contain cadmium, a mineral which the body cannot use and which is closely associated with high blood pressure. Cadmium is also found in superphosphate, a fertilizer used in food production; we can therefore ingest cadmium through the food chain without knowing it, as well as by smoking cigarettes.

Blood pressure does not remain constant; it varies. It is lower when the body is resting and it tends to rise during physical exertion, emotional disturbances or after the use of stimulants, (e.g. coffee, alcohol etc.). Stress, either physical or emotional, causes a temporary rise in blood pressure. When stress becomes a feature of everyday life the blood pressure is raised over a longer period and tends to stay that way. Relaxation is essential to reduce tension and control blood pressure. When the body is tense, the nerves are set on edge; anger or emotional upset causes blood vessels to contract and blood pressure to rise.

Genetic factors also play an important role. A person's genetic make-up determines how prone he is to develop high blood pressure. Some people are unfortunate from a genetic viewpoint and it is not uncommon for high blood pressure and circulatory trouble to run in families. Nevertheless, it is by no means impossible to reduce the influence of genetic weaknesses in this area. It has been clearly demonstrated that Australian aboriginal people and New Guinea nationals, living in their natural environment before the influence of white men, had very low blood pressure and practically no circulatory disease. However, when introduced to the white man's diet of salt, fat, sugar and refined carbohydrates, their blood pressure rose to equal that of the white man with the resultant circulatory disorders.

This clear observation indicates that diet is the major cause of high blood pressure and its related diseases. A diet high in salt, fat, sugar and refined carbohydrates increases the production of cholesterol which clogs up the arteries and reduces their diameter, alters the electrolyte balance causing the muscular walls of the arteries to contract and creates mineral deficiencies, particularly magnesium deficiency. This causes death of muscle cells, followed by coronary thrombosis or myocardial infarction. High blood pressure can not only be prevented by a sensible diet but also dietary support during treatment can have a critical influence on recovery.

There is not doubt that the two major factors influencing high blood pressure are genetic factors and diet. We cannot do anything about our genes, but we can do a great deal to adjust our diet and lifestyle to overcome this disorder and open the door to a fuller, richer and longer life.

1

What is High Blood Pressure

In order to understand what high blood pressure is and how it may develop, it is necessary to first consider how the blood circulates through the body.

The centre of the circulatory system is the heart which functions as a very sophisticated pump. As the heart muscle contracts the blood is distributed into the blood vessels known as arteries. The force at which it is carried to various parts of the body depends partly on the pressure at which it leaves the heart and partly on the elasticity of the blood vessels carrying it.

There are therefore two factors which contribute to the maintenance and control of the blood pressure. At each heartbeat the blood is pumped into the arteries with a certain force which can be measured. At the time of the beat the pressure is at its highest point. This is known as the systolic pressure. As the heart relaxes to gather strength for the next beat the blood pressure falls to its lowest level. This is known as the diastolic pressure. It is easy to confirm this on yourself by feeling the pulse in the wrist. It goes up and down in rhythm with the beats of your heart.

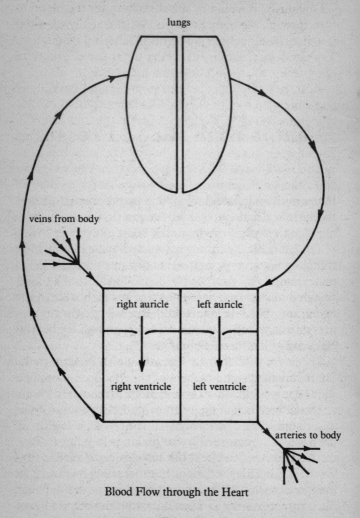

Blood Flow through the Heart

Fig. 1

Obviously, it would be unsatisfactory for the blood to flow through the body in spurts. What is really required is a nice, steady, even flow. This is achieved through an ingenious mechanism that relies upon the elasticity of the arteries which will be discussed shortly.

First, however, it is helpful to undertand how blood flows in and out of the heart. The heart consists of four compartments. On the right side is the right auricle (sometimes known as the atrium), which is the receiving chamber for blood from the body. The auricle is connected via a valve to the right ventricle. The only exit from the right ventricle leads to the lungs so that all blood from this compartment must go through the lungs where it is aerated to take up oxygen.

From the lungs, the freshly aerated blood is returned to the left auricle which is connected through a valve to the left ventricle. Blood leaves the left ventricle to be distributed to all parts of the body.

Blood vessels that bring blood to the right side of the heart are called veins. Those that carry it away are known as arteries. The flow of blood through the heart is shown diagrammatically in figure 1.

Let us look now at the sequence of blood flow as the heart contracts or beats:

1. During the heart's relaxed stage (diastole), oxygen-depleted blood from the veins of the body flows into the right auricle. At the same time, the left auricle fills up with oxygen-rich blood from the lungs (see figure 2).

2. A natural pacemaker built into the right auricle fires eletrical impulses causing both auricles to contract simultaneously. At the same time, the valves between auricles and ventricles open, allowing the blood to flow into the ventricles (see figure 3).

from body   from lungs

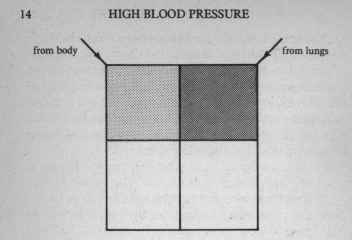

Fig. 2

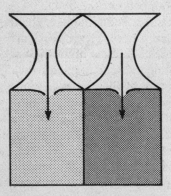

right ventricle   left ventricle

Fig. 3

3. The next stage is the pumping one in which electrical signals from another node cause both ventricles to contract simultaneously. This forces oxygen-depleted blood from the right ventricle into the lungs. Oxygen-rich blood from the left ventricle is pushed out into the main artery called the aorta from where it disperses to all parts of the body. The valves close to ensure there is no back-flow into the auricles (see figure 4).

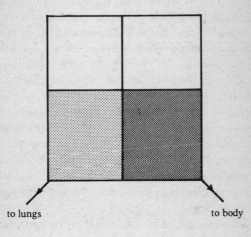

to lungs   to body

Fig. 4

4. After the contraction of the ventricles, the heart relaxes allowing the auricles to fill with blood and the whole sequence starts again.

This sequence of events takes places about seventy times a minute when the body is relaxed. During exercise, the whole process quickens up.

In one day the heart distributes 1,440 gallons of blood. A high proportion of this is supplied to the heart muscle itself via the coronary artery. The requirements of the heart for oxygenated blood are high. Hence the drastic consequences when the blood supply to the heart fails.

Arteries and Veins

It has been calculated that there are some 60,000 miles of blood vessels in the adult body. They begin at the heart and serve every organ and tissue. The main artery leaving the left ventricle of the heart is the aorta, a thick-walled vessel of about one inch diameter. This branches into smaller arteries which get progressively smaller and narrower, eventually ending in tiny hair-like tubes invisible to the natural eye and called capillaries.

Capillaries are the only blood vessels that are permeable to liquids and gases. They are also the means by which oxygen and nutrients are fed to the tissues, and waste products from the tissues are exchanged.

These capillaries progressively widen to give rise to veins which act as the collecting blood vessels of the body. Eventually, they join up and bring deoxygenated blood to the heart.

The arteries and veins differ in their construction and this reflects their different functions. All arteries are constructed in the same way; each has three coats or layers and is not unlike a rubber hose-pipe.

The outer layer is tough and fibrous to give the blood-carrying inner tube protection. The middle coat is a ring of muscle which has the power to contract and expand under the influence of special nerves. When this artery muscle contracts, the tube is narrowed. Relaxation causes the diameter to increase, allowing more blood to flow along it. Hence, as an artery constricts, the pressure increases and as it relaxes, the pressure drops. This property of elasticity is very important in controlling the blood pressure. The inner coat of the artery is smooth so that blood can slip and glide through it easily.

Not all arteries have the same amount of elasticity. The pulse in the wrist or neck can be felt to go up and down with the heartbeat. In the smaller arteries of the muscles, the eyes and the brain, however, there is no pulse because the blood flow is steady.

Arteries have to withstand high pressures, so they are thick-walled and muscular. Veins, however, are not subjected to these high pressures, so they do not have to be of such robust construction. These are therefore thin-walled and have no muscle layer. They contribute to blood flow through a system of valves which ensure that the blood moves off towards the heart. When these valves do not function correctly, the veins sag as blood falls back, and the end result is the condition known as varicose veins.

The blood vessels that feed the organs and tissues far removed from the heart are known as the peripheral blood circulation system. We shall see later how this system contributes an important function in the control of blood pressure.

How Blood Pressure is Measured
The measurement of blood pressure is a valuable diagnostic tool and the technique is a simple one.

A flat rubber bag with two outlets is wrapped around the patient's upper arm. One outlet connects to a column of mercury. The other is attached to a rubber bulb via a valve so that the pressure within the bag can be increased and decreased at the will of the observer.

The detector, in the form of a stethoscope, is then placed over the chief blood vessel of the arm at the inner fold of the elbow. The heartbeat is easily heard and the bag around the upper arm is inflated by pumping the rubber bulb until the point is reached when the air pressure in the bag is just sufficient to overcome the arterial pressure. At this stage no sound is heard.

As the amulet is gradually deflated by careful manipulation of the valve, the heart sound is heard again and the first sign of this indicates the systolic pressure.

With further decompression the thudding character of the sounds is replaced by soft, murmuring qualities which, in time, are replaced by clear sounds. With still further decompression the sounds disappear and this is the point of the diastolic blood pressure.

Blood pressure is always expressed as two figures but it is the second, lower figure that is the more meaningful in diagnosing high blood pressure. No doctor will be content with just one reading and the technique is likely to be repeated twice or three times.

The average adult figure for systolic pressure is between 120 and 130 millimetres of mercury. For the diastolic phase, the average reading is between 75 and 85 millimetres. A diastolic pressure of greater than 90 millimetres is usually indicative of high blood pressure.

Mild hypertension describes the condition when the diastolic pressure is between 90 and 95 millimetres of mercury. It is often first discovered accidentally during the course of a life insurance or routine medical examination. The patient seldom complains of any symptoms and usually nothing is done, except to measure the blood pressure regularly to ensure that it is not showing any tendency to rise.

A diastolic blood pressure of between 105 and 120 millimetres of mercury is described as moderate hypertension. The common symptoms are headache, heart discomfort (particularly on exercise) and breathlessness. Often these are improved by simple dietary treatment and advice.

When the patient is overweight, dietary restriction to cause a loss of 1 to 1.5kg per week will often relieve the symptoms and bring about a significant reduction in blood pressure. This is essential as the chances of developing coronary heart disease whilst suffering from hypertension are greatly increased if the individual is also obese.

The advice given is aimed at allowing patients to organize their lives so as to avoid emotional stress and excessive physical activity. This will be dealt with in more detail later.

When reduction in weight and a change in lifestyle are not sufficient to lower the blood pressure, drug therapy is often called for. These include drugs aimed at reducing the pressure (hypotensive drugs) and those that simply remove excess water from the body (diuretics). Cutting down the intake of common salt is often as effective as the drug therapy.

Severe hypertension, with diastolic pressures over 120 millimetres of mercury, is usually treated with a combination of the measures used in moderate hypertension. These will be dealt with later in a discussion of how drugs may bring down the blood pressure.

How High Blood Pressure Involves Other Organs
Do not imgaine that a blood pressure reading is like the

measurement on a speedometer or the figure on some electronic instrument. The actual figures only express what is happening during the few seconds the reading is taken. Blood pressure changes from day to day and even hour to hour, depending upon physical and emotional activities. Such changes however are only temporary and the blood pressure usually falls back to normal.

As you grow older, the reading of the systolic pressure tends to rise and this is normal since it is due to the condition known as hardening of the arteries, associated with old age. Hence, it is often the arteries which are first involved in the development of hypertension.

Hardening of the Arteries

Hardening of the arteries is a degenerative disease. Degenerative ailments are usually slow in their onset as well as being painless until well advanced.

The medical term for hardening of the arteries is arteriosclerosis. It is characterized by a thickening and decrease of elasticity of the walls of the artery, resulting in a narrowing of space through which the blood flows, known as the lumen. As the diameter of the lumen decreases, a greater force is required to push the blood through it. The heart responds by increasing the pressure of its beat. The result is high blood pressure. At the same time, in arteriosclerosis the elasticity of the artery walls is lost because of the deposition of unwanted material in the two inner layers of the blood vessels. The important contribution of the elastic property of the artery walls in maintaining blood pressure is removed, so a greater strain is thrust upon the heart itself which responds by increasing the power of its beat. The result is sustained high blood pressure.

Hardening of the arteries may be caused by the deposition of mineral salts which may be likened to the 'furring-up' of hot water pipes in areas of hard water supply. It may also be a result of the deposition of fats and fatty substances such as cholesterol which, as well as causing the artery walls to lose their elasticity, can also slowly build up to result in an actual blockage.

The consequence of arteriosclerosis, whether caused by mineral deposits or fats, is the same: possible rupture of the artery wall. This is not surprising when it is considered that the arteries are partly obstructed by deposits when it is considered that the same volume of blood must now go through narrowed and less elastic blood vessels; there is bound to be an increased likelihood that these vessels will rupture under stress.

There are four groups of arteries extremely liable to rupture in such circumstances. They are in the heart, in the kidneys, in the brain and at the back of the eyes. Bleeding from the back of the eyes is fairly common in very high blood pressure but it serves as a protection to the arteries in the brain because such bleeding lowers the danger pressure at the brain, even if only temporarily.

Inspection of the interior of the eye is therefore of prime importance in any examination by your doctor when he is considering the possibility of hypertension.

Inspection of the Eye
Inside the back of the eyeball is the retina, a light-sensitive layer of cells that may be likened to the film inside a camera. The retina is covered with a rich network of arteries and veins. By means of an opthalmo-scope, an instrument which allows both illumination and inspection of the eye, a doctor is able to assess the

health of the veins and arteries of the retina.

The beauty of this technique is that the interior of the eye is the only place in the body where the arteries can actually be observed. In this way, the doctor can see whether they are thickened or have ruptured or have any other abnormality. He is able to judge whether the high blood pressure is having any effect upon them.

The eye may be regarded as part of the brain (it has been called 'the window into the brain') so that any damage to its blood vessels may reflect possible risk to the brain arteries. Examination of the eye is important as it enables the doctor to continuously monitor the condition of the blood vessels in anyone suffering from hypertension.

The Kidneys

The kidneys represent two of the target organs which the doctor keeps under constant watch when he is treating high blood pressure. When the urine is centrifuged, the solids that are spun to the bottom of the tube can be examined microscopically and they indicate the extent of kidney damage induced by high blood pressure.

If the kidneys are regarded as filtering units of the blood, the force at which this is pushed through the filters determines what appears in the urine. Protein, for example, is not usually found in urine because the filtering units of the kidney (the glomeruli) will not let such a large particle through. When the blood pressure is high however, the glomeruli partly collapses under the increased force upon them and allow the blood proteins to filter through. The amount of protein, its type and appearance in the urinary deposit tells a doctor a lot about the state of the kidneys and particularly about any damage induced by increased blood pressure.

Other examinations involving the kidneys in the hypertensive patient include injecting a harmless chemical dye into the blood stream. This dye is concentrated in the blood vessels of the kidneys so that they become visible on X-ray. Thus any changes by an increased blood pressure will become apparent to the expert eye.

The Heart

This is the most important of the target organs which have to be considered in the person suffering from high blood pressure. Tests are available for examining heart function and estimating the pumping power of its four chambers.

Its electrical reactions recorded on an electrocardiogram (ECG) will indicate the health of the heart muscle itself. At the same time, the expert will be able to assess the efficiency of the electrical stimulation of heart muscle, which determines the power and frequency of the heartbeat.

An X-ray of the chest will reveal whether the heart muscle has become thickened to adjust to the high blood pressure. Enlargements of one or more of the heart's chambers is indicative of any potential failure of its pumping capacity. This will tell the practitioner whether his treatment of high blood pressure is correct and will indicate any future complications that may arise.

The diagnosis of high blood pressure is thus not just a matter of an isolated measurement, although this may be the first indication that something is amiss. The consequences of raised blood pressure are more important than the fact that it exists. Once a patient has been diagnosed as hypertensive, the target areas mentioned above become the main cause of concern to the doctor and his mode of treatment depends upon his assessment of how they are affected.

Symptoms of High Blood Pressure

These include severe pounding headaches, especially in the back and sides of the head, a feeling as though a band was being tightened around the head; poor memory, head noises, shortness of breath, insomnia, nervousness, dizziness and sometimes the appearance of blood in the urine are among the other symptoms experienced. Swelling of the ankles is also a common feature of high blood pressure. It is due to retention of water and is known as oedema. When the puffy part is pressed with the finger the resulting dimple is retained for some seconds. If it is not oedema, the tissue regains its original shape immediately.

It must be remembered, however, that such symptoms occur only with a sustained high blood pressure. All of us have transient rises in blood pressure in situations of danger, excitement, anger and stress because this is nature's mechanism for generating an adequate supply of blood to the brain. Similarly, at times of exercise as in athletics and other sports, the muscles require more blood and oxygen which is supplied by an increased pressure. Once the emergency or exertion is over the blood pressure reverts to normal. In the hypertensive patient this is not the case.

The long-term consequences of high blood pressure include strokes, heart attacks, kidney failure and respiratory problems.

Strokes vary in their intensity, depending on how widespread their effect is. A minor stroke occurs when the pressure is sufficient to burst a tiny artery in the brain causing a small localized haemorrhage. The effects may be no more than a little difficulty in speech, memory or in walking for a day or two. Sometimes the individual recovers completely.

The second type of stroke is induced by a blockage in an artery of the brain, usually caused by a small blood clot. What happens is that the part of the brain supplied by that blood vessel becomes depleted of blood and the loss in supply of nutrients and oxygen causes that area to die. If the part affected is of minor importance and is restricted to any small area, the symptoms will be similar to those described for a small haemorrhage.

When the stroke is more intense, however, the results are indeed serious. There is often prolonged unconsciousness and sometimes the eyes, mouth and head are pulled to one side. The stentorian breathing greatly alarms relatives, as well it might — some 64 per cent of serious strokes are fatal.

As the patient recovers consciousness, he or she is often left paralyzed on one side, a condition known as hemiplegia. The arm is often rendered useless, being permanently bent into the side and the fingers are turned towards the palm. The leg is often affected, while speech is reduced to a few scarcely articulated words. The crowning humiliation is that the victim's bowels and bladder are no longer under his control.

The arteries supplying the heart may also suffer as a consequence of high blood pressure. The aorta can develop a weakened area of wall known as an eneurysm which may rupture under increased pressure. The consequence is usually a massive haemorrhage that is invariably fatal.

More likely, however, is a thickening of the coronary arteries produced by deposition of fat. If the closure is gradual, the condition is known as *angina pectoris,* a disease marked by intense pain in the vicinity of the breast bone and which may travel down the left arm and sometimes into the jaw. Sometimes the fat is deposited inside the artery to such an extent that it completely blocks the blood supply and hence the supply of oxygen to the heart muscle. If this happens, a coronary thrombosis results which may be fatal. With only partial blockage, the individual may eventually suffer a heart attack from which he subsequently recovers.

What is without doubt is that high blood pressure will eventually cause enlargement of the left ventricle of the heart. This eventually causes congestion of the lungs since you will recall that the left auricle sends blood to the left ventricle from where it is then distributed to all parts of the body. When the left ventricle is unable to do this, a back pressure builds up which forces blood back to the left auricle and hence to the lungs. At the same time the right ventricle is inefficient in supplying blood to the lungs, complete oxygenation cannot take place and the result is breathlessness.

There may also be a serious effect upon the kidneys. The renal arteries which supply blood to these organs become hardened and thus less efficient. Bio-chemical waste products in the blood that are normally passed out in the urine are retained. The result is a vicious circle that tends to sustain the high blood pressure.

Hence a very high blood pressure is more likely to give rise to the more serious strokes and heart attacks. A mild brain haemorrhage or thrombosis or a partial coronary thrombosis should be regarded as a warning that there is more to follow. It also indicates that the individual should be changing his or her lifestyle. Dietary considerations are of prime importance in this respect and we shall see later in the book how self-help in the form of sensible eating and specific supplementation with certain nutrients can prevent blood pressure and even treat it.

Types of Hypertension

In a minority of patients, blood pressure is very high. This is called malignant hypertension. The heart, kidneys, eyes and arteries elsewhere in the body are quickly affected. There is a vastly increased risk of a vascular accident (i.e. thrombosis or burst vessel), so fast and vigorous treatment is required. This treatment is beyond the capacity of the normal individual and skilled medical assistance is essential. What a person can do, however, is to reduce the chances of malignant hypertension developing by a sensible diet and lifestyle.

In the majority of cases of high blood pressure (about 80 per cent), clinical investigation does not reveal a cause for the condition. This is known as essential hypertension. Treatment is aimed at alleviating the symptoms and it is essential hypertension that is more likely to respond to natural treatment.

The reason for the development of the remaining cases of hypertension resides in detectable conditions in other parts of the body. The most common is kidney disease followed by glandular dysfunctions. Pregnancy also predisposes to hypertension although this usually disappears once the baby is born. When high blood pressure is secondary to other diseases, it usually reverts to normal once the underlying condition is successfully treated.

2

The Causes of High
Blood Pressure

There are several contributing causes in this condition. It is not enough to say that 'hardened arteries is a condition of old age'. Hardened arteries is often a cause of old age in people who should be in the prime of life.

People living under natural conditions, eating simple, natural foods, do not have high blood pressure. It is unknown among native races. Investigations have been made into why coronary disease and high blood pressure are almost unknown among New Guinea natives who are noted for their good health, strength and fine physiques. The blood pressure of the natives is about the same as young Australians, but it never increases with age, as it does in Australia. Doctors practising in New Guinea cannot explain why the natives, both in the hills and on the coast, are so free of these diseases.

It should be noted that the native diet comprises sweet potatoes, taro, yams, bananas, nuts, and in recent years, sugar cane. Coastal natives eat fish as well, but all these foods are wholesome, natural and unprocessed. All contain their full quota of vitamins and minerals, yet the doctors affect to be surprised that the New Guinea natives are practically free from heart ailments and high blood pressure, which rank as number one and number three 'killers' among Australians. High blood pressure is essentially a degenerative condition, due to our civilized diet and our so-called civilized way of life.

Diet is enemy no. 1, as far as high blood pressure is concerned. The diet of the sufferer from high blood pressure consists, and has consisted for some years, of a mixture of foods which contain a great excess of protein, starch and sugar, in addition to an assortment of de-vitalized, demineralized foods, all of which may leave harmful deposits in the system.

Being too much for the kidneys to eliminate in the urine, uric acid salts (urates) may be deposited on the arterial walls, thus reducing their elasticity and restrict-ing the circulation of the blood.

But worse, his or her diet includes too many animal fats which often leave cholesterol on the inside walls of the blood vessels. It is cholesterol plus uric acid deposits and minerals which silt up the arteries, bringing about the condition known as hardening of the arteries, and the high blood pressure that results from it.

The Dangers of Stress Must not be Overlooked

Some of the causes and consequences of high blood pressure may be related to stress. Stress may be physical or mental, but it is difficult to qualify it. There is the stress associated with physical danger and this should be considered to be both normal and natural. It takes many forms such as life-threatening situations, business problems, worry about the health of oneself or a near relative or simply the strain of everyday living. What happens is that the heart beats more forcibly and rapidly. Glands such as the thyroid and adrenals respond by increasing the secretion of their active hormones. The brain's requirements for blood also increase.

However, one of the fundamental reactions to danger, in addition to these, is a rise in blood pressure. The heart is responding to the increased demand for blood from the brain and muscles by supplying it faster. Such a response may be regarded as one of nature's defence mechanisms and is a perfectly natural one. Once the danger has gone, the body reverts to normal. It is when these various reactions, including blood pressure, persist that problems arise. Thus the kind of stress that keeps the blood pressure up for many months or even years will eventually result in a condition that must be treated.

Those who drive long distances at sustained speeds on motorways have been found to have raised blood pressure over periods of several hours. Little wonder then that constant stress can contribute to a permanently raised blood pressure.

Diabetics and Hypertension

In maintaining health it is vitally important that blood sugar levels are stabilized within a relating narrow range. Such close control is achieved by the hormone insulin which is produced by the gland known as the pancreas.

Those suffering from diabetes have lost this control, either because they do not produce enough insulin or because it has failed in its function. The sustained high blood sugar that results gives rise to increased blood pressure. Sometimes the first noticed sign of diabetes is hypertension.

The relationships between high blood pressure and a

high blood sugar level reflects what may happen when an individual is on a diet rich in refined sugar. The constant high sugar concentration being absorbed into the blood stream can, eventually, not only induce a consistently increased blood pressure, but may exhaust the powers of the pancreas to produce insulin.

Overeating is a recognized cause of obesity which, in turn, often gives rise to diabetes, resulting ultimately in hypertension.

Hypertension and the Menopause

During the menopause, the blood pressure is often higher than normal. This is partly a consequence of aging in the individual, since hardening of the arteries, resulting in loss of elasticity, is a feature of the older female.

Other changes occur during the menopause, notably those associated with the decreased production of female sex hormones. Stress may give rise to emotional upsets and these can also induce high blood pressure. Hypertension, however, is probably a result of the influence of both factors. What is nevertheless apparent, is that correct dietary principles can be used to treat all the symptoms of the menopause, including that of hypertension.

Defective Kidneys and Hypertension

Just as the heart pumps all the blood through the circulatory system every seven minutes, so it also passes through the kidneys in the same amount of time.

The function of the kidneys is remarkably intricate. These two little organs weighing less than eight ounces each, consist of an amazing network of tiny filter tubes which in total measure 280 miles!

The body's entire blood supply passes through these tubes every few minutes and it is the function of the kidneys to filter out of the blood all the uric acid waste matter and expel it from the body via the bladder. Now, it will be appreciated that if the diet overloads the kidneys, certain serious things happen:

a. The kidneys themselves become affected. Those 280 miles of sensitive filter tubing become silted up.

b. The blood is not properly purified.

c. The unexpelled uric acid salts are deposited along the walls of the arteries and veins.

In short, blood pressure is heightened and kidney trouble is manifested. Either of these conditions is serious, but when both are experienced together, the outcome is generally fatal.

The mechanism of kidney involvement in producing high blood pressure is a complicated one. Thickening of the renal (kidney) artery by deposition of fat, hardening of this artery by deposition of salts or simple blockage by a thrombus all reduce the oxygen supply to these vital organs. This, in turn, stimulates the kidneys to produce an enzyme called renin, an excess of which causes high blood pressure.

Other kidney diseases that can produce similar effects are inflammation of the filtering units (glomerulone-phritis), retention of water (hydronephrosis), cysts and cancer of the kidney. Later, I shall examine how an excessive intake of common salt induces high blood pressure via its effect upon the kidneys.

Tobacco Smoking and Hypertension

Though we have not listed tobacco smoking as a main

cause of blood pressure, there is no doubt that the weight of clinical and laboratory evidence is strongly againt it as just one more factor in contributing to high blood pressure.

Dr Logan Clendening, in his book, *The Human Body*, writes: 'Tobacco has quite measurable effects. Principally these are a constriction of the blood vessels, through their muscular coats, and a rise of blood pressure.'

Dr Emil Bogen, Professor of Public Health, University of Cincinnati, and author of numerous scientific and biochemical studies with regard to tobacco, has expressed these opinions: 'The circulation responds to nicotine with a marked vaso-constriction or narrowing of the blood vessels. This constriction of the blood vessels is followed by a rise in the blood pressure. The various instruments used in recording the blood pressure show changes in the systolic reading after even a few cigarettes have been smoked. There is positive evidence, too, that smoking induces secretion of the adrenal glands, which, in turn, promotes a rise in the blood pressure.'

U.S. Army Medical Corps officers conducted a study of six men smoking cigarettes, all habitual smokers who inhaled. The experiment showed temporary constriction of the arteries after smoking. The pulse rates returned to normal five to fifteen minutes after the cigarettes, but vascular restriction of the arteries persisted for half an hour to an hour, in some cases much longer.

The famous Mayo Clinic recently conducted an experiment to ascertain the effects of cigarette smoking upon blood pressure. The test was made with a number of persons suffering from hypertension and others with a normal blood pressure. These persons were required to rest until the blood pressure and pulse rate reached a basal level. After this, each was required to smoke a cigarette of standard type and strength, the blood pressure and pulse rate being checked during and a few minutes after completing the smoke.

The test proved that a considerable rise in blood pressure followed the smoking of the first cigarette, with a further rise after the second was smoked. A careful reading was made in each case and the figures faithfully recorded. The smokers commencing with a normal blood pressure showed an increase of 21.1 systolic and 13 diastolic, while those whose pressure was already above normal recorded figures as high as 31.5 and 18.4 respectively.

Tests made by Dr W. J. McCormick, Toronto, Canada, reveal that one cigarette cancels out 25 milligrams of vitamin C in the body. The daily adult requirement of vitamin C is approximately 250 milligrams, so that ten cigarettes can entirely deplete the body of its supply of this most important vitamin. Very little vitamin C is stored, and it must be taken daily.

Of course, people smoke for a reason and this is because nicotine is a soothing and tranquillizing agent. However, against it is the fact that cigarettes also cause metabolic changes, in addition to those mentioned above.

When smoke is inhaled into the lungs, the resins in tobacco irritate the linings of the bronchii, the main tubes leading into the lungs, as well as the delicate tissue of the lungs themselves. The result is chronic bronchitis and the well known 'smokers' cough'. Any cigarette smoker throws an extra burden on his heart and circulation since inhaled smoke must deprive the system of air and hence oxygen.

It has been argued that nicotine might relax the blood pressure through its soothing effect, but in no way does this compensate for its deleterious effects on the heart and blood vessels. In cases of hypertension, a cigarette smoker is at greater risk than a man who does not smoke cigarettes. Those smokers who do not inhale tobacco smoke, namely cigar and pipe smokers, may be at less risk than the cigarette smoker, but it must be remembered that absorption of harmful constituents can still take place directly through the mouth. By not smoking at all, we can at least remove one factor that can contribute to high blood pressure.

Dietary Factors and Hypertension

It is generally agreed by nutritional scientists and doctors that dietary factors must rank as the first consideration when looking for the causes of high blood pressure. These factors, either singly or in combination, are now regarded as:

1. Excessive protein in the diet. Too much protein causes a viscous (thickened) blood stream.
2. Excessive intake of animal fats causing cholesterol to be deposited on the walls of blood vessels.
3. Devitalized food which leads to glandular imbalance.
4. Too much salt in the diet.
5. A high calorie intake causing excess body weight.
6. Specific vitamin and mineral deficiencies that induce nervous complaints.
7. Inefficient elimination of toxic substances present in and formed from the food eaten.

1. *Excessive Protein in the Diet*
Protein foods are meat, fish, eggs and cheese. There is

also a small amount of protein in bread, milk and other foods, but the chief protein foods of general consumption are eggs and meat.

Protein foods form the building material of the body and they repair waste. Since the average man and woman doing average physical work only consume (i.e. use up), about three ounces of tissue daily, all the protein food required to replace this dead tissue is an equal amount; or, allowing for non-assimilated matter such as gristle in meat, say three to five ounces daily.

If more protein is eaten than is needed for tissue replacement and repair:

a. The protein may cause a viscous, gluey or thickened blood stream. Meat fats are rich in cholesterol; the more viscous a fluid is, the more resistant it is to flow, and the greater the pressure required to force it through a narrow tube.

The heart is given a heavier task to pump this thickened blood stream and, if subjected to overstrain for years, it becomes tired and defective in function.

b. Protein foods are almost wholly digested in the body. There is very little residue which finds its way into the large bowel for elimination. But what it does do is to charge the blood stream with several acid urates.

If the kidneys cannot cope with the task of eliminating these poisonous uric acid wastes from the blood, the whole circulating mechanism — that is to say, the arteries and veins — become gradually silted up with them. In time, they form a hard, stony deposit on the arterial walls, thus robbing the walls of their elasticity and giving the blood a narrower system of arteries and veins to flow through.

It will be seen, then, that blood which is being pumped

through the circulatory system at the rate of sixty gallons an hour, must inevitably put greater pressure on the narrowing walls in its effort to travel to all parts of the body.

Now the function of protein foods is to replace dead cell tissue. It must be understood that every part of the body consists of cells, and that these cells, which are composed of protein, are constantly dying and are being replaced and repaired by new cell tissue. The person who suffers from blood pressure cannot get a sound grasp of the problem which confronts him until he understands the far-reaching effects of excess protein in the diet.

The end product of protein metabolism is a compound called urea that is usually dispersed through the kidneys. Any excess protein will give rise to high levels of urea in the blood and this in itself may cause an increase in blood pressure. Usually though, the kidneys rid the body of excess urea quite efficiently.

When the kidneys are diseased, they lose the ability to dispose of the blood urea and the result is a permanent increase in blood pressure. Two features of kidney disease are a high blood urea level and hypertension.

Dr William Howard Hay, the celebrated nutritional and medical scientist, and director of the East Aurora Sanatorium has written as follows on the cause of blood pressure in his book, *Some Human Ailments*: 'If there is one distinctly American disease, in this land of different-iated maladies, this one is sure to be, by unanimous consent of the entire medical profession, the condition described as cardiac-vascular-renal disease, or in plain English, degeneration of the heart, arteries, and kidneys, one disease with three heads, one degenerative condition with three expressions in combination.

'The number of those who die from some complication induced by this three-headed organic degeneration of heart, arteries and kidneys, and the number suffering in lower efficiency from the same cause, can never be computed, and if this were possible the total would be staggering indeed.

'In a close observation of many hundreds of cases of blood pressure, hardening arteries, degenerating kidneys, dilating hearts, in a private and sanatorium practice covering the past thirty years, I have not seen one single exception to the rule that an excess of protein is behind every case, the average being well over ten times as much protein as Chittenden says is necessary to repair body waste . . .'.

Dr Howard Hay goes on to say that bad cases of blood pressure are tremendously benefitted, and the milder ones more so, by a protein-free diet for a time, following a general cleansing of the system of its toxic debris.

2. *Excessive Intake of Animal Fats*

Dietary fats are of two types, roughly divided into those derived from animals and those derived from vegetables. Dairy products supply the animal variety.

Fats obtained from animal foods are solid and hard with a waxy appearance; think of butter, lard and beef tallow. On the other hand, fats derived from cereals, seeds and vegetables are liquids such as wheat germ oil, sunflower seed oil and soya bean oil.

The reason that some fats are hard and others are liquid oils (with some in between) is that they all differ in their degree of saturation. All fats contain the elements carbon, hydrogen and oxygen and their physical appearance depends on the ratio of carbon atoms to hydrogen atoms.

When the carbon atoms in a fat are combined with the maximum number of hydrogen atoms, the fat is called unsaturated. Unsaturation can occur to varying degrees. If the carbon atoms are almost saturated, i.e. they lack any two hydrogen atoms, the product is mono-unsaturated. When many carbon atoms are deficient in hydrogen atoms the result is an oil which we call poly-unsaturated. These oils are found in non-animal foods.

A good balanced diet will supply all three types of fat, saturated, mono-unsaturated and poly-unsaturated. However, it is the proportion of these three kinds of fat that determine how healthy a diet is. When there is a high proportion of saturated and mono-unsaturated fats problems may arise because the body does not have the ability to convert these fats to the poly-unsaturated variety. The body needs poly-unsaturated fats (or oils) for health and the only source of them is the diet.

It is relatively easy for a chemist to convert liquid poly-unsaturated oils into hard fats by chemically adding hydrogen to saturate the carbon atoms. This is known as hardening of the oils and is the process used to produce hard margarines. What he is doing is taking health-giving, nutritious vegetable oils and changing them to the hard fats just like those found in animal products which, as shall be discussed later, can contribute to ill health leading to high blood pressure and heart complaints.

The so-called soft margarines are produced by partial hydrogenation (or hardening) of the oils to give a product that retains much of the poly-unsaturated nature of the starting material. Alternatively, they can be made by blending a small amount of fully hardened fat with a large amount of the unprocessed vegetable oil. The result in either case is a soft margarine that is an excellent source of the health-giving poly-unsaturates but, of course, neither will be the same as the original untouched oils.

The type of fat we eat determines, to a large extent, how likely we are to develop diseases such as hypertension and coronary heart disease. In the so-called developed nations of the world, the national diet has changed considerably over the last few decades. Less starchy foods such as potatoes and bread are eaten while consumption of refined sugars and fat has increased. This fat has been mainly of the saturated kind which we have seen comes from animal foods and dairy products.

Many studies which have looked at mortality and the development of certain diseases in primitive and rich communities throughout the world have shown that the deaths from coronary heart disease, associated with hypertension, appear to increase with higher intakes of saturated fats. At the same time, these intakes are associated with high blood cholesterol levels; the higher the diet is in animal-derived fats, the higher the blood cholesterol level. High blood cholesterol in turn appears to be a factor in inducing fatty deposits in blood vessels which we have seen is an important contributory factor in producing high blood pressure.

Hence, saturated fatty acids may be asserting their deleterious effect via cholesterol and we shall now look at the role of this fatty substance in contributing to the development of hypertension and eventually coronary heart disease.

The Role of Cholesterol

What is cholesterol? It is a fatty substance that is a constituent of all animal fats and is particularly high in brains, kidneys, liver and other offal, egg yolk, butter, cream and all fatty meats. Plant products, vegetables and fruits are essentially free of cholesterol.

Cholesterol is also in an essential body constituent. It is an important component of fatty myelin sheath. This is the natural insulating material that surrounds and protects nerves and has a similar function to the plastic or rubber surrounding an electric cable. Cholesterol is also the precursor of the sex hormones and stress hormones which the glands of the body produce.

Cholesterol is also the starting material in the production of vitamin D. The action of sunlight on the skin converts a substance in the skin (produced from cholesterol) into this essential vitamin. Therefore, when sufficient sunlight falls on the skin enough vitamin D is synthesized so the dietary intake of this vitamin under these conditions becomes less important.

The bile acids which are essential components of the digestive system are also made from cholesterol. Since bile acids are needed for the efficient digestion and absorption of fats, it is evident that cholesterol, another fat, has a most important function.

In appearance, cholesterol is a hard, waxy substance which means that once it is deposited in blood vessels and tissues it creates a blockage that is difficult to move. There are body mechanisms that usually prevent this by keeping cholesterol mobile and in solution. It is when these systems break down or when blood cholesterol levels are excessively high that the scene is set for the abnormal deposition of cholesterol.

The most important substances that contribute to this control of cholesterol are the poly-unsaturated fatty acids and a complex compound called lecithin. Lecithin itself contains poly-unsaturated fatty acids as well as two important members of the vitamin B complex known as choline and inositol. All of these components combine to keep cholesterol dissolved in the blood and so prevent its being deposited on the walls of blood vessels.

Much of the cholesterol in the body is not present as such but is combined with fatty acids. When these fatty acids are of the poly-unsaturated type which we have seen are contributed by vegetable oils and lecithin, the resulting combination is much less liable to be deposited in the wrong places. When cholestrol is combined with the hard fats obtained from animals, the resulting combination is more insoluble and more difficult to keep in solution.

The importance of lecithin and of its B vitamins, choline and inositol, in controlling fats is easily demonstrated in experimental rats. When these animals are deprived of these essential dietary constituents, they die of fatty liver. Post-mortem examination reveals all of the essential organs literally saturated with fat. If such animals are treated with lecithin before death, the condition can be reversed and the fat is shifted from the liver and essential organs, redistributed throughout the body and eventually burned off as energy.

Lecithin and poly-unsaturated fatty acids are only two of the dietary factors which can help control fat and cholesterol in the body. However, lecithin can be made, to a certain extent, within the body, assuming that sufficient poly-unsaturated fatty acids and the B vitamins, choline and inositol, are present in the food. A healthy supply of lecithin or its constituents must therefore be contributed from the diet.

It has been shown that cholesterol is an essential body constituent, but that at high concentration it can cause problems. There are, however, two sources of cholesterol. The first is the diet but this represents only a minor contribution. Most of the body's cholesterol is made by synthesis within the body itself.

In a healthy individual, when a lot of cholesterol is eaten, the body responds by making less. If not much cholesterol is eaten, as for example in the case of vegetarians, there is more synthesis to keep body levels up. When things go wrong and high blood cholesterol levels result, the reasons are usually found in excessive body synthesis. This in turn can be controlled by dietary means through lecithin and other nutrients or, in extreme cases, using drugs. Dietary intake of cholesterol appears to assume less importance in controlling really high levels of blood cholesterol.

There is no doubt that cholesterol as a major cause of heart disease and high blood pressure, is not theory alone. We have only to examine the eating habits of various nations to prove it.

Dr J. Keys of U.S.A. did a lot of research on this question. In Italy, in 1951, his studies showed that the Italian diet contained only half as much fat as the American diet and the death rate from heart and blood pressure diseases in that country was only one-third as high as the American rate at that time.

Incidentally, the fat calories of the Italian diet consist largely of olive oil — a vegetable oil containing lecithin; and lecithin, as discussed, dissolves or emulsifies cholesterol.

When Germany occupied Norway in World War II, the fat calories in the Norwegian diet were greatly reduced — and so was the incidence of heart and blood pressure diseases.

Drs A. R. P. Walker and J. Higginson of Johannesburg, South Africa, measured the cholesterol levels of certain African tribes. They found that the Bantu, who get only fifteen per cent of their calories from fats, had a little cholesterol in their blood. In a series of 224 autopsies on Bantu males fifty to seventy years old, they found only one death from coronary disease.

The rice and fish eating Japanese live on one of the lowest fat diets in the world. Did this mean that the Japanese heart was one of the healthiest? Prof. Noboru studied 10,000 autopsies and personally examined 1,007 hearts. Incidence of seriously diseased coronaries in Japan proved to be about one-tenth of that in the United States or Australia.

3. *Devitalized Food and Glandular Deficiency*

The third cause of high blood pressure is the amount of devitalized food present in the diet — white bread, processed breakfast foods, white sugar, tinned foods, 'instant foods', over-cooked vegetables, biscuits, pastry, jam, and those attractive but devitalized concoctions bought at the delicatessen. From the point of view of nutrition, the foregoing are impoverished foods which cannot adequately nourish living bodies. Their vitamin or mineral value is usually reduced considerably.

If you read the Science of Life book *Liver Ailments*, you will see that where the diet is lacking in essential vitamin and mineral values, the endocrine glands fail to function efficiently. They fail to secrete their various hormones into the blood stream, and the whole body chemistry is upset.

The other effects of eating the kind of devitalized food referred to is that it further loads the blood stream with uric acid wastes, which lower the level of general health, break down kidney function, and silt up the circulatory system.

Devitalized food is generally regarded as being deficient in vitamins and minerals and this deficiency in itself may contribute to high blood pressure. Another factor is often missing from processed and refined foods. This is dietary fibre, the indigestive part of the diet, lack of which is now believed to contribute to many of the so-called diseases of civilization, among which is numbered hypertension.

As long ago as 1937, Dr C. P. Donnison had established, through a wide survey of a group of Kenyan tribes, that essential hypertension was virtually absent among these people in 1929. Similarly in the West, Dr E. H. Hipsley in 1953 concluded that a dietary fibre protected against toxaemia of pregnancy and hypertension.

One of the leading proponents of dietary fibre, Dr H. C. Trowell, gave his opinion in a symposium in 1977, stating that the tendency towards hypertension in susceptible people is decreased by energy-food fibre (e.g. bran) and also by the higher potassium content of unprocessed and unrefined cereals. Devitalized foods lack both fibre and potassium. When rats were given starchy foods rich in fibre they showed less tendency to high blood pressure than those given starchy foods without fibre.

Another observation was made by Drs H. C. Trowell

and D. Burkitt in 1977, reporting on a study of African tribesmen. Once these people switched to a Western-type diet, the first new disease to appear was hypertension. This was followed by disease of the brain blood vessels. Obesity, constipation and haemorrhoids emerged next, to be followed by diabetes and heart disease. Hence, diseases that were unknown in these people when they lived in the natural state appeared only when they switched to devitalized food lacking in vitamins, minerals and dietary fibre.

4. *An Excess of Salt in the Diet*

A relationship between salt and hypertension has been suspected since 2000 B.C. when the Chinese Emperor Huang Ti wrote: 'Hence, if too much salt is used in food, the pulse hardens.'

Studies carried out on individuals from different countries, from the East and the West, have shown a broad correlation between salt intake and blood pressure. Japanese who lived in Japan had diets containing low salt levels. When they emigrated to the U.S.A. and switched to Western diets, their salt intake increased and so did their blood pressure.

Studies by Dr L. K. Dahl in the U.S.A. (*American Journal of Human Nutrition*, 1972) looked at Americans who were divided into three groups: those who habitually added salt to their food at table; those who added it only when necessary and those who never added salt at table. He found that the greater the salt intake, the higher the blood pressure that developed.

These results have been challenged by others but they were recently confirmed by similar studies in the U.K. and reported in *The Lancet* (May 1981). To assess long-term salt intake, each individual was asked whether he or she added salt to the following foods; fish, vegetables, salads, potatoes and eggs. Points were given for each positive reply and when the results were calculated there was a definite correlation between the amount of salt eaten and the blood pressure. High salt intake increases the blood pressure. The research workers involved concluded that a restriction of salt intake would reduce the incidence of hypertension and the accompanying diseases affecting the blood vessels of the heart and brain.

An important point to emerge is that salt restriction will prevent the development of high blood pressure but may also help reduce it when hypertension is already present.

It must also be remembered that the part of salt that induces hypertension is sodium. This mineral is also present in baking powder and mono-sodium glutamate and therefore these sources of sodium must also be curtailed when seeking a low-sodium diet.

5. *High Calorie Intake and Overweight*

Cause no. 1 dealt specifically with the effects of excess protein, but the effects of overeating in general should not be overlooked. One might say that the whole Australian dietetic tradition is to overeat. According to life insurance statistics, this is the reason why six out of ten people are overweight by the age of forty. And from then onwards most people go on adding pounds to their bodies. The end result of this overeating tradition is disastrous to health.

Every meal we eat requires blood for its digestion. The bigger the meal, the larger amount of blood required. In other words, the bigger the meal the harder the task of the heart, kidneys and circulatory mechanism.

It is this excessive feeding tradition which, carried on over a lifetime, partly results in one person in every four dying of heart failure, long before his time. It is this excessive feeding tradition which contributes to the fact that one person in every ten succumbs to a paralytic stroke. It is this excessive and indiscriminate feeding tradition which will kill over one million Australians now living. One person in every ten is doomed to die of it — unless he changes over to the nutritional principles outlined in this book. The human body runs far more efficiently on half the amount of food usually eaten, provided it is the right kind; it must be remembered that the heavier the meal, the greater the blood pressure.

Incidentally, the typical blood pressure type — virile with prodigious energy and drive — is apt to overdo everything. He usually eats heartily and excessively. He attacks a meal as he attacks a problem — aggressively.

The dangerous effect of excess weight was stressed by Professor Edward H. Rynearson, associate professor of medicine at the Mayo Foundation of U.S.A.: 'Thousands of Americans are literally eating themselves to death,' he said in the course of an address to the 28th annual meeting of the American College of Physicians.

'The fatter people get, the shorter their lives will be,' said Professor Rynearson, adding that persons who over-eat expose themselves to diabetes, high blood pressure, heart disease, kidney ailments, arthritis of the legs, hip or spine, gall bladder disease and varicose veins. 'Their bodies are overworked by overeating', he said, and the only way to cut them down to size is dieting. 'There's never been a patient in the history of medicine who couldn't reduce if he had the will power', Professor

Rynearson added. A heart encased in an envelope of fat is seriously impeded in its action.

6. *Specific Vitamin and Mineral Deficiencies*

There is no doubt that a healthy nervous system depends upon adequate quantities of vitamins and minerals being made available to it. The nervous control of the heart also requires these nutrients and the stimulation of these nerves, in turn, determines the output and force of the blood leaving it. Deficiencies of some vitamins and minerals can therefore indirectly induce high blood pressure.

If a serious deficiency of these factors affects the average man, how much more will it affect the typical blood pressure type — the restless, worrying, hard-working, aggressive type, who drives himself and everybody else?

Without adequate calcium, the B-complex vitamins and vitamin C, such a person scarcely knows what it is to relax. But once these deficiencies are made good, a calmer demeanour gradually asserts itself. The restlessness is modified, and the worrisome aggressiveness gives way to more constructive expenditure of precious energies.

As Dr R. Harrison has pointed out, 'a diseased or starved nervous system causes chronic spasmodic contractions of the muscle walls of the arteries'.

The metabolism of calcium is intimately related to that of magnesium since, for every atom of calcium outside a nerve cell, there is a complementary atom of magnesium inside it. This arrangement allows nerve impulses to be carried along a nerve rather as the electric current travels along a wire.

In magnesium deficiency there are thus malfunctions between the transmission of nerve impulses and the contraction of the muscles they are controlling. The symptoms are high excitability, tremor and convulsions with behavioural disturbances such as depression. This is why magnesium has been termed the natural tranquillizer since simple supplementation with it overcomes such symptoms.

These symptoms are often the prerequisites of hypertension. As magnesium deficiency worsens, the heart and blood vessels become affected as the blood pressure increases. Eventually, the blood vessels of the brain constrict and the result is often a stroke.

The Need for Vitamin B_6

H. A. Schroeder, M.D., of the Washington University Medical School, St. Louis, U.S.A., writing in *The Journal of Chronic Diseases*, says that a lack of vitamin B_6 in the diet of monkeys produces hardening of the arteries and in laboratory rats it causes high blood pressure.

'There is evidence,' he adds, 'that the whole process takes place in the blood vessels of these animals very much as it does in those of men.'

The reason for this lies in the conversion of an amino acid called methionine to another known as homocysteine. Homocysteine is a toxic compound that is quickly converted to an important amino called cystathionine in a reaction that requires vitamin B_6.

In the absence of vitamin B_6, toxic levels of homocysteine build up in the body and the result is hypertension due to a thickening of the blood vessels by fatty deposits.

Some unfortunate individuals are born with the inability to convert homocysteine to cystathionine and the result is high blood pressure and atherosclerosis at an early age. In fact, anyone with atherosclerosis invariably has low blood levels of vitamin B_6 and high blood levels of homocysteine. This vitamin must therefore be considered essential in preventing some causes of high blood pressure.

Further evidence is provided by a study of 46,000 women who had taken the contraceptive pill for at least five years. This form of contraception is notorious for inducing vitamin B_6 deficiency. The study revealed that these women had an incidence of high blood pressure, heart and blood vessel disease and leg thrombosis some ten times greater than matched females not taking the 'Pill'. The evidence is thus highly suggestive that lack of vitamin B_6 is a contributory factor in the high incidence of these conditions.

The Need for Choline

Choline is a member of the vitamin B complex and also forms part of the complicated structure of lecithin. Body levels of choline come from two sources. It is eaten in the diet but can also be synthesized by the body itself. Despite the apparent adequate availability of choline, however, there is evidence that it can be deficient in some individuals.

In prolonged low levels of choline in the body the result can be high blood pressure. When it was given to a group of patients suffering from hypertension, the typical symptoms of palpitations, dizziness and headaches disappeared within two weeks of treatment. Blood pressure was reduced to normal levels at the same time.

The mechanism of this action is not known, but it is

3

The Control of Hypertension with Vitamins and Nutrients

We have seen that hypertension is not a disease in itself but is of prime importance in the development of coronary heart disease, strokes and kidney disease.

The other risk factors are cigarette smoking and dietary-induced high fat levels in the blood. The presence of excessive cholesterol, which is also a fat, again constitutes a high risk of precipitation on the walls of blood vessels, leading to thrombosis.

Cigarette smoking increases the risk of fatal heart disease twice or three times, but heavy smokers under the age of 45 have a ten to fifteen times greater risk than non-smokers. Stopping smoking rapidly reduces this risk.

Slight to moderate hypertension greatly increases the risk of a coronary attack. A man aged 35 with a blood pressure of 160 systolic/100 diastolic reduces his life expectancy by sixteen years. Diabetic patients have a much increased risk of fatal coronary heart disease.

First let us examine how the type of fat in the diet can help us reduce the prospect of high blood pressure and even lower it, once established.

How Dietary Fat Can Help

The influence of dietary fat on our health is best illustrated by an example from Japan, as already mentioned in Chapter 2.

Japan is a modern, industrialized, stressed, well nourished and heavily smoking society with no problem of coronary heart disease. The Japanese have a concentration of fats in the blood much lower than that of those who live in the West but normal when compared with other low-risk populations.

This can be explained by their habitual healthy diet which is low in saturated fat and cholesterol but includes a high intake of poly-unsaturated oils. It is also characterized by relatively little protein from land animal sources; more seafood than meat; little dairy produce and a high intake of cereal, pulses and other vegetables. They thus consume little fat and what they do consume comes mainly from poly-unsaturated vegetable sources. The carbohydrate eaten is of the complex, poly-saccharide type as in starches rather than the refined sugar kind which is known to contribute to high blood pressure development.

In Japanese who have migrated to the United States and who have changed their dietary habits to that of typical Americans, fat and cholesterol levels in the blood increased. The result was development of arteriosclerosis which led, in due course, to the same incidence of coronary heart disease as in the indigenous population.

A further pointer to the importance of low-saturated fat in the diet is provided by a study of an isolated tribe of bushmen in north-west Botswana.

The level of cholesterol in the blood of these bushmen averaged 120mg or 100ml. Compare this with the 150 to 250mg per 100ml that is considered the normal range in adults in the U.K. Although these people do eat some meat provided by the wild buck, this animal has no fat around it and what little fat it does have is of the poly-unsaturated type.

More than half of the energy in the diet of the bush-men is provided by vegetable foods. The largest single item in their diet is a locally grown nut which is a good source of protein but which has the particular attribute of a high content of linoleic acid. This same health-giving poly-unsaturated fatty acid is also found in high concentration in sunflower seeds, safflower seeds, corn or maize, wheat germ, soya beans and most of all in oil of Evening Primrose. Any society therefore has access to these important poly-unsaturated vegetable oils and partial replacement of saturated fats with these oils must be the first dietary consideration of anyone wishing to avoid hypertension and its consequences. Needless to say, the bushmen do not suffer from any degree of high blood pressure. Unlike those in Western society, blood pressure levels of the bushmen actually decrease with age.

The Official Attitude

Twenty official committees drawn from many countries throughout the world have made recommendations regarding dietary intakes of various foods in attempts to reduce the incidence of high blood pressure and coronary heart disease.

It is generally agreed that fat of all kinds should con-tribute only between 30 and 35 per cent of the energy requirement. In many Western countries, fat accounts for 50 and 60 per cent of an individual's energy requirements. When it is considered that one gram of fat yields nine calories which is more than twice those provided by a similar weight of carbohydrate and protein, it is essential in most diets to reduce the amount of fat. This means that for an average female taking 2000 calories per day, the total fat intake should not exceed 74 grams which is just over 2½ ounces. A man who requires 3000 calories per day should not eat more than approximately 3½ ounces of fat.

With only two exceptions, all the committees recommended an increased intake of poly-unsaturated fatty oils at the expense of the saturated kind. This means a switch from animal and dairy fats to the vegetable oils, remembering, however, that the total fat intake should not exceed 35 per cent of daily calories.

A committee drawn from New Zealand and one from the U.K. were both of the opinion that all fat intakes should be reduced but no guidance to the actual reduction was given.

In general, it was recommended that the type of fat eaten should be fifty per cent saturated and fifty per cent poly-unsaturated. It was almost unanimously agreed that the intake of cholesterol-rich foods should be curtailed so that only between 300 and 400mg per day of cholesterol was in the diet.

Strong recommendations were made that sugar intake should also be reduced and that energy should be obtained from complex carbohydrates that are found in whole cereals and vegetables rather than in sweetened foods.

The principles laid down in these official recommendations will help to do two things. First, blood and tissue fats will be reduced; second, blood cholesterol will be lowered. Both of these beneficial effects are of paramount importance in preventing the development of high blood pressure and in lowering this in those already suffering from it.

How Cholesterol May Be Reduced

a. *By Means of Diet*

The first consideration in reducing blood cholesterol is to control the intake of those foods where it is present. The richest sources are (mg per 100g found in brackets): butter (280); cod-liver oil (850); hard cheeses (160-190); soft cheeses (140); cream (100-130); eggs (463 but none in egg white); whole milk (10); brain (2360); heart (150); kidneys (410); liver (320).

Poultry provide much less cholesterol, with chicken contributing only 90mg per 100g (3.5 ounces) and turkey with merely 15mg per 100g. Most fish supply only moderate amounts of cholesterol (usually about 60mg per 100g), but beware of other seafoods. Lobster (145), oysters (230), shrimps (150), and caviar (490) must be regarded as substantial sources of cholesterol.

Fruits, vegetables and cereals may be regarded as substantially free from cholesterol as are seeds and the oils obtained from them. Such foods can be eaten liberally by anyone seeking to refrain from a high cholesterol intake.

b. *By Means of Lecithin*

Lecithin is known as an 'unsaturated fatty acid', and it has the property of breaking up cholesterol by mixing with it and keeping it finely divided so that it becomes emulsified and circulates freely instead of congealing and solidifying, causing great harm to the arteries.

When man began to refine his cereals, particularly wheat, he removed not only lecithin from his food, but also vitamin E, the B group of vitamins, and certain minerals that are essential to health, including iron.

Animal fats are a poor source of lecithin and the enormous increase in heart disorders and high blood pressure cases clearly indicates the serious lack of essential vitamins and minerals in the daily diet.

Arteriosclerosis, or hardening and narrowing of the arteries, is now a common symptom in people of the fifty and over age bracket. Why has this symptom become so general? The answer given by one large and authoritative school of medical opinion is, because of the refining and cooking of foods. It comes about this way: cholesterol is present in most animal fats. It is especially rich in egg yolk, brains, kidney, butter, cream and meat fats, but also present in egg yolk and in other foods, is a substance called lecithin.

Lecithin, when present in foods with cholesterol, prevents cholesterol from depositing on the arterial walls. Lecithin, as we have seen, has the capacity of emulsifying cholesterol and keeping it soluble in the blood stream.

In the last half century, serious and significant changes have taken place in the processing of food. This processing which the various fats and oils go through before they appear on the grocery shelves, destroys the lecithin content, but leaves the cholesterol.

Hydrogenated fats, for instance — the shortenings used in pastry and for frying — do not contain lecithin, for it has been destroyed in the hydrogenation process. Margarine, processed cheeses and other foods are treated by the hydrogenation process with the same result. Hydrogenation is a method of treating edible fats and oils, whereby hydrogen is forced through them in a chemical process. This processing converts soft fats and oily substances into a semi-solid consistency, enabling them to be cut with a knife, and thereby greatly facilitates handling, packeting and selling, but it also greatly reduces their lecithin content. Hence the cholesterol in foods becomes deposited on the arterial walls, and high blood pressure is the result.

Lecithin contains a vitamin of the B group called choline, whose particular function it is to transport and utilize cholesterol and other fats within the body. It also contains inositol.

Tests carried out at the Toronto (Canada) Medical School by Dr C. H. Best, have demonstrated that young animals kept on a diet low in choline, later developed high blood pressure and that their abnormal blood pressure is proportionate to the severity and the duration of this deficiency of choline. Choline deficiency also caused severe haemorrhages in the tubules of of the kidneys and eventually nephritis (Brights' Disease) was produced in these test animals.

Inositol, another B-complex vitamin, also aids in the body's utilization of fatty substances.

Lecithin is not confined to vegetable foods and is found in substantial quantities in eggs for example. However, when it is present in animal-derived foods its fatty acid content reflects their source and tends to be of the saturated type. This lecithin may not be as effective as that derived from vegetable sources such as the soya bean since the presence of poly-unsaturated fatty acids in vegetable lecithins appears to confer on these a better cholesterol-lowering action.

Similarly, if the diet contains a high intake of poly-unsaturated fatty acids, these will be incorporated into the lecithin also provided by the diet. Hence, by cutting down on animal fats and increasing the intake of vegetable lecithin, either by diet or by supplementation, it is possible to ensure that the powerful emulsifying action of lecithin on cholesterol in the blood and organs is maintained.

The beneficial action of vegetable lecithin in reducing blood cholesterol levels has been amply demonstrated by many researchers but the pioneer in the field is Dr Lester Morrison, a heart physician from Los Angeles. He chose patients who had consistently high blood cholesterol levels and in whom all other cholesterol-lowering treatments had failed. All these patients had high blood pressure and this, combined with their increased blood cholesterol levels, made them high risks for heart attacks and strokes.

All the patients were given a tablespoonful of pure soya lecithin granules three times a day with meals. At the end of three months, eighty per cent of the patients were found to have significantly reduced blood cholesterol levels averaging 156 milligrams per 100cc blood, which means a reduction of 41 per cent. Blood pressure was also found to be lower at both the systolic and diastolic levels.

The significant features of this trial, and indeed many similar ones, are: (i) reduction in blood cholesterol; (ii) reduction in blood pressure and (iii) complete lack of side effects. In addition, all those patients who responded to lecithin felt better, fitter and were able to go back to a normal lifestyle.

c. *By Means of Nicotinic Acid*

The B vitamin, nicotinic acid, has been shown to have the ability to reduce blood cholesterol levels. However, in the form of nicotinamide, although it has all the other attributes of the vitamin, this has no effect upon blood cholesterol.

A short-term trial studying the property of nicotinic acid to reduce blood cholesterol in those patients with high levels was reported from the Mayo Clinic in 1956. A total oral dose of three grams of nicotinic acid given daily over two weeks reduced the blood cholesterol to normal levels in 72 per cent of those tested. Increasing the dosage of nicotinic acid to four to six grams per day lowered the blood cholesterol in the remaining 28 per cent.

A longer-term study carried out over eleven years at the Dartmouth-Hitchcock Medical Centre in New Hampshire indicated that lower intakes of nicotinic acid could also lower the blood cholesterol but at a slower rate. A relatively low dose of 100mg of the vitamin after each meal, followed by an increased intake of one gram after every week, reduced the blood cholesterol in all patients by an average figure of 25 per cent. This decrease was maintained whilst therapy with nicotinic acid continued, even though the intake of the vitamin was reduced to only 200mg per week. There were no significant side effects with this treatment, the most serious being a slight flushing in some patients.

Nicotinic acid does not appear to act alone in this respect. There is evidence that the mineral chromium combines with nicotinic acid and the resulting complex is the active factor in reducing blood cholesterol.

Studies carried out in Britain have indicated that nicotinic acid also has the property of lowering blood fats (known as triglycerides) at the doses used in reducing blood cholesterol. It is as effective in this respect as the drug clofibrate. The big difference, however, is in the safety of the two treatments. Nicotinic acid showed no serious side effects. The drug clofibrate has recently been discontinued in the U.K. because of its toxicity.

Nicotinic acid reduces blood fats by inhibiting their synthesis. At the same time it competes with and prevents the release of free fatty acids which combine with cholesterol. Hence, this property of reducing blood fats combined with its ability to lower blood cholesterol levels contributes indirectly to its anti-hypertension effect by preventing the narrowing of arteries by fatty deposits.

Nicotinic acid also exerts a more direct action in reducing high blood pressure. It causes the minor blood vessels to dilate and this, in turn, makes the flow of blood easier. The end effect is that, against this decreased resistance, the heart does not have to work as hard and a lower blood pressure results.

d. *By Means of Vitamin C*

Modern research suggests that vitamin C (ascorbic acid) has an important function in controlling blood cholesterol and fat levels in man.

The leading researcher in this field is Dr Emil Ginter of the Institute of Human Nutrition Research, Bratislava, Czechoslovakia. His conclusions, reached after many years research, are these:

(i) The lower the vitamin C level of a person, the higher are the cholesterol and blood fat levels.

(ii) Treating diabetics, who usually have high blood cholesterol, with 500mg vitamin C per day reduced their levels to normal.

(iii) Those with high cholesterol levels not associated with any specific disease also responded to 500mg vitamin C per day with a reduction in both fat and cholesterol levels.

(iv) Vitamin C at this level had no lowering effect on the blood cholesterol of those with normal values.

(v) Hence, vitamin C reduces blood cholesterol concentration and then maintains it at normal levels.

The reduction of blood cholesterol is achieved by vitamin C in a simple, safe and effective manner. It does so by increasing the rate at which cholesterol is converted into bile acids which are then excreted. This represents the main source of cholesterol excretion in the body. Blood fats are also reduced by vitamin C but its method of action here is not as well documented as that of cholesterol.

It may be highly significant that one of the early signs of an impending stroke is the haemorrhage of the tiny blood vessels under the tongue and these also appear in vitamin C deficiency. When 500mg of the vitamin is taken daily, these signs disappear and the tongue resumes its normal appearance.

Deaths from coronary heart disease and strokes increase in numbers during cold weather when the need for vitamin C is highest, but intake is often lowest. This observation could be explained by the protective action that the vitamin appears to have on these conditions according to Dr Constance Lesley of the Wakefield

Group of Hospitals. Vitamin C may help prevent heart attacks, strokes, deep-vein thrombosis and athero-sclerosis through its fat- and cholesterol-controlling function described by Dr Ginter.

We know that fat and cholesterol deposition is only one factor in increasing the risks of these conditions. Stress, diet, smoking and alcohol may also contribute. Yet separate studies have shown that all of these may lower the vitamin C levels in the body and increase the body's requirements. Perhaps, therefore, vitamin C deficiency is the prime factor responsible for increased blood levels of fats and cholesterol which we have seen may be the fore-runners of high blood pressure and its consequences. An adequate intake of vitamin C of the order of 500mg per day is a sensible way of reducing the chances of these blood-related diseases.

Reducing High Blood Pressure with Other Vitamins

a. *Vitamin E*
The great effectiveness of vitamin E in the treatment of heart diseases and high blood pressure is shown in the outcome of researches by Drs Evan and Wilfred Shute and a research scientist named Floyd Skelton, of the Shute Foundation for Clinical and Laboratory Medicine, London, Ontario, Canada.

Vitamin therapy opens up a new era in the treatment of cardiovascular diseases (diseases of the heart and circulatory system). The great increase in these diseases in the last few years convinced Dr Evan Shute that the increase was due primarily to the refining of foods.

The folly of refining flour by the removal of the wheat

germ, the polishing of rice, the growing of vegetables with artificial fertilizers, the picking of fruits before they are sun-ripened — all these practices deprive human beings of their ordinary supply of vitamin E.

Speaking of the effect of vitamin E treatment in cardiovascular diseases, Dr Evan Shute made this claim: 'There must be failures in any treatment — nothing in medicine is perfect. But we have not learned of a single failure. The percentage of success is remarkable.'

High blood pressure cases require 100 milligrams of vitamin E daily for four weeks, 120 milligrams daily for the next four weeks, and so on, increasing at the rate of 20 milligrams daily per month until a maximum dosage of 300 milligrams daily is being taken, or until the symptoms of high blood pressure disappear. Where there is thyroid trouble, however, no more than ten milligrams daily of vitamin E should be taken, until this gland disorder has responded to suitable therapy.

Nature's curative processes are slow. One is obliged to apply the new principles consistently and intelligently for some months. In the average case, there is marked improvement in a few months, and, finally, the reward of intelligent perseverance is that blood pressure should return to normal and all symptoms of it disappear.

b. *Inositol*

Inositol is a member of the B-complex group. It is present in lecithin and so may contribute to the fat- and cholesterol-lowering effect of this nutrient with its concomitant effect of reducing high blood pressure. However, like choline, inositol appears to have beneficial effects on the heart and blood vessels in its own right.

In 1949, Drs I. Leinwand and D. H. Moore (*The American Journal*) found that three grams of inositol daily lowered the fat and cholesterol levels in the blood of atherosclerotic patients. Their high blood pressures were also reduced. In mild hypertension, with no apparent cause, the use of one gram of inositol, given morning and night, produced a gradual lowering of the blood pressure. Another important benefit conferred by this amount of inositol was a sedative effect at night which is often appreciated by those suffering from high blood pressure with its accompanying symptoms.

c. *Bioflavonoids* (*Vitamin P*)

Rutin is one of the bioflavonoids and is obtained as a by-product of the milling of buckwheat. It has a beneficial effect upon the blood capillaries and the other minor blood vessels which, in turn, help to control the blood pressure.

For many years, buckwheat has been used in herbal medicine as a means of reducing high blood pressure. The does required is between two and four grams per day and the herb must be taken continuously to maintain a normal blood pressure. This amount of herb contains about 150mg of rutin. Hence, a similar benefit is obtained by taking rutin itself in tablet form. Bioflavonoids are non-toxic and this quantity of rutin is perfectly safe to take.

Bioflavonoids are also present in hawthorn berries which are a traditional remedy for high blood pressure. However, hawthorn is also a heart stimulant and great care must be exercised in controlling its dosage.

Magnesium and High Blood Pressure

Low blood magnesium levels are often a feature of the disease known as arteriosclerosis (hardening of the arteries) and usually result in disturbances of heart rhythm. In experimental animals, Dr J. Rigo of Semmelweis Medical University, Budapest, found that a high intake of magnesium lowered high blood pressure. Rats that had an induced high blood pressure developed abnormal aortas but on treatment with magnesium, both conditions were reversed.

The presence of magnesium may also be a reason why people who live in hard-water areas have less chance of developing heart disease than those living in soft-water areas. Hard water contains this mineral but soft water does not and it has been calculated that drinking water can contribute significant quantities of minerals to the diet when they are present. There is also evidence of lowered magnesium concentrations in the heart and other tissues of those people dying of heart disease associated with hypertension.

Taking supplementary magnesium is simple. Dolomite tablets (two with each meal) provide the mineral along with calcium in the correct proportions. For best absorption, take magnesium as the amino acid chelate, either alone or in the form of Amino Acid Chelated Dolomite.

The richest food sources of magnesium include wholemeal bread (but not white), soya beans, all nuts, shell fish, dried peas and lentils, brown rice, figs, dates and dried brewer's yeast.

Diet and Vitamin Dosage

The following diet and vitamin supplementation will

ensure an adequate intake of the vitamins that we have discussed and which are essential to help keep the blood pressure down to normal levels. Supplementary vitamins may be necessary to actually reduce the blood pressure when this is high and those have been discussed in the individual sections above.

Trace minerals, as we have seen, are also extremely important in maintaining a normal blood pressure and these will be supplied in the kelp tablets recommended. However, there may be felt to be a need for additional chromium and selenium in view of recent research into these trace minerals. Yeast is an excellent source of chromium and it can also be taken as the amino acid chelate.

Selenium is best taken in conjunction with vitamin E since the vitamin and mineral function more effectively in the body as a combination. There is no direct evidence that high blood pressure is related to a lack of selenium, but there is no doubt that it does have a protective action upon the heart. It is therefore prudent to ensure that when vitamin E is taken, it is accompanied by selenium since any positive action of vitamin E in maintaining a normal blood pressure and a healthy heart can be increased in the presence of this trace mineral. A daily supplement of selenium of between 75 and 100 micrograms should suffice, but it is essential that it is taken in the organic form, preferably incorporated into yeast.

Before Breakfast: A glass of diluted orange juice (no sugar) and one or two vitamin C (250mgm) tablets; 1 vitamin B_1 (10mgm) tablet; 1 B-complex tablet; 1 kelp tablet (for its iodine content); 2 calcium tablets (white) and half your daily dosage of vitamin E.

Breakfast: Three dessertspoonsful of wheat germ with

milk. You can have the cereal by itself (with milk) or with a grated apple, or you can follow it with a plate of stewed apricots or prunes, peaches or grapes.

Morning Tea: Cup of weak tea or a diluted fruit drink (orange, grapefruit, orange and lemon, pineapple or tomato juice).

Before Lunch: 1 B₁ (10mgm) tablet; 1 B-complex tablet; 1 vitamin C (250mgm) tablet; 2 calcium tablets (white); 1 kelp tablet and 1 lecithin capsule (250mgm). All can be taken together.

Lunch: One of the following meals: two apples and 3 oz (75g) of unprocessed cheese, (no bread); a green leaf salad, with grated carrot, grated beetroot, grated apple, parsley, etc., and a glass of milk; a plate of fruit and a glass of milk (Four ripe peaches, for example, and a glass of milk is an ample — and excellent — meal for a blood pressure sufferer.); 1 lb (½ kilo) of grapes.

After Lunch: 2 vitamin A and D capsules.

Afternoon Tea: Cup of weak tea or a diluted fruit drink.

Before the Evening Meal: 1 B₁ (10mgm) tablet; 1 B-complex tablet; 1 vitamin C (250mgm) tablet; 2 calcium tablets (white); 1 kelp tablet; 1 lecithin capsule, and the second half of your vitamin E dosage for the day.

Evening Meal: If you had fruit and cheese for lunch, now is the time to have your large salad. In winter, precede the salad with hot soup, but make the soup fresh each day and do not overcook it. In summer, the salad may be followed by fruit, a little custard or ice cream. As a change, a plate of steamed vegetables may be served with cheese sauce.

After the Evening Meal: 2 vitamin A and D capsules. When on the road to recovery, a small grill or fish may be added — no more than twice per week.

Before Bed: Check up on the vitamin aspect of your diet for the day, and make good any omissions. A glass of diluted fruit juice means an easier sleep than tea or coffee.

4

The Control of Hypertension by Dietary Means

The following seven corrective principles should be followed to alleviate the condition of hypertension:

1. Reduce such protein foods as meat and eggs to the minimum and, *during the period of treatment, cut them out altogether*.

2. Cut down on all foods, especially foods rich in animal fats. Eat lightly — and rightly. Base your meals on those suggested on pages 91-94.

3. Cut out all dead and devitalized foods. (See taboo list on page 81).

4. Cut out all pepped up and stimulating food and drink.

5. Base your diet on the 80-20 principle for sound health; that is to say, see that your daily food intake consists of approximately four-fifths of fruit, salads, vegetables and milk and only about one-fifth of starch and protein foods.

6. Make it a policy to control all emotional upsets. 'They are not worth the candle' with the ever-present danger of a stroke.

7. See that you get adequate amounts daily of all the essential vitamins — A, B-group, C and E as well as calcium and kelp (to keep the thyroid gland in health). All are of vital importance, and vitamin E especially.

The amazing results from vitamin E in all heart and blood pressure cases is one of the triumphs of modern science. *The American Journal of Physiology* carried an article some years ago by Drs K. L. Zierler, D. Grob and J. L. Lilienthal describing experiments which showed that vitamin E dissolves blood clots in veins and arteries.

Meat Eating Fallacy

Now let us deal with the foregoing principles in more detail:

1. During the period of treatment, the high blood pressure sufferer should cut out meat and eggs altogether.

As I have already mentioned, these proteins are one of the chief factors in causing a gluey, sticky, viscous blood which puts an unfair strain on the heart and increases the tension on the arterial walls. The tradition that meat is essential for strength is a fallacy. The British people are meat eaters by tradition. But there are examples of physically powerful — and far healthier — people who eat meat only occasionally. One such race is the Hunzas of Northern India.

According to Sir Robert McCarrison, an eminent medical scientist who spent some years among the flesh-abstaining natives of that locality, the Hunzas are 'an example of a race unsurpassed in perfection of physique and in freedom from disease in general, whose sole food consists of grains, vegetables and fruits, with a certain amount of milk and butter, with goats' meat only on feast days'.

During nine years of medical practice among these people, Sir Robert McCarrison found that men of seventy years of age had the youth and vigour of European men of thirty. During his years among the Hunzas, he never came across one case of cancer, colitis, high blood pressure, gallstones, appendicitis or stomach ulcer.

In an address entitled *Blood Pressure, What Affects It?* given by Dr A. Hunter to an association of U.S. medical men, he stated: 'Taking the population of the United States as a whole, I believe that a better adjusted diet, with less animal protein food, would result in a lower blood pressure, a longer life, and a greater capacity to carry out the obligations of life.'

Professor E. V. McCollum, of Johns Hopkins University, a scientist of world repute, has written this about meat: 'All the evidence from both animal experimentation and human experience supports, in a manner which cannot be broken down, the viewpoint that meat is not necessary in the human diet.'

The Interallied Council of Physiologists during the Second World War said: 'It is not thought desirable to fix a minimum meat rations in view of the fact that no absolute physiological need exists for meat, since the protein of meat can be replaced by other proteins of animal origin — such as those contained in milk, cheese and eggs — as well as by proteins of vegetable origin.'

Wheat germ and brewers' yeast, also powdered skimmed milk, are all excellent sources of protein that have none of the disadvantages of meat.

The Art of Eating Less
High blood pressure subjects usually have a history of

hearty appetite. They have eaten well but not wisely. It cannot be too strongly emphasized that their safety from a deadly illness which menaces them lies primarily in diet.

Surely, sufficient medical authority has been put forward to convince readers of the evils of excess protein. We are now obliged to emphasize equally the dangers of overeating in general.

The average blood pressure sufferer is a 'good doer', and a great deal of what he eats builds up tissue fat and blood. If he values his life — and his sanity — he will resolve to eat much less, eat very lightly and eat far better in future; that is to say, he must select his food with more intelligence. He must quickly learn that for high blood pressure sufferers, a salad is a far, far wiser meal than meat and vegetables, followed by a dessert.

He must cultivate the all-fruit-meal habit, such as two apples or three or four ripe peaches or a pound of grapes, or a dish of stewed fruit. An all-fruit meal is a better lunch for blood pressure sufferers than sandwiches, a grill, an omelette, or corned beef, fish or cold chicken. The raw salad vegetables — grated carrot, grated beetroot, grated apple, lettuce leaves, parsley, celery sticks, tomatoes, ripe sliced bananas and sliced pears, etc., supply the blood with most of the essential vitamins and minerals.

These foods purify the blood, detoxicate the system, reduce the viscosity (stickiness) of the blood, and thus reduce blood pressure. These three factors are fundamental to any cure or any improvement in the condition.

The high blood pressure sufferer must get rid of the erroneous notion that a salad of an all-fruit meal as part of his daily diet will 'sap his strength'. On the contrary, his health, his energy, and his strength will improve amazingly as his blood pressure is reduced by sound nutrition. Just as unsound nutrition has been the main cause of his blood pressure, so will sound nutrition correct it. The raw salad vegetables and fruits are revitalizing. The more vital your food, the more vital your health.

Foods on the Taboo List

The blood pressure sufferer should completely eliminate the following dead, devitalized foods from his diet:

Salt
Sugar
White bread
Meat fats
Processed breakfast foods
Strong tea
Pepper
Condiments of all descriptions
Biscuits and cakes
Confectionary of all kinds
Tinned meats and other tinned foods
Re-heated or re-cooked foods
Corned meats
All desserts other than fruit or stewed fruit
Jam
Sausage meats
All puddings
Most packeted and 'instant' or ready prepared foods
Processed cheese
Fried foods
Coffee
Soft drinks

The above 'foodless foods' are notorious for causing most of the ills from which the body suffers. They are responsible for saturating the tissues with acid end-products and for silting up the vascular (circulatory) system with uric acid deposits. They are a cause of glandular malfunction, which slows up the whole governing mechanism of the body. In short, the long-term effect of these 'foodless foods' is homicidal. Now that you know the truth about them, to continue using them is suicidal.

Foods to be Cut Down

The following foods should be drastically reduced: all kinds of meat, fish, eggs, alcoholic beverages, bread, potatoes, butter and cream.

If the patient's condition is serious, he would be advised to cut the above food out of his diet for the duration of the treatment, and thereafter partake of them very sparingly.

A Warning

The blood pressure sufferer should be warned that the foregoing somewhat sudden changes in his diet will have rather disturbing physical and psychological effects.

Nature does not adjust herself quickly, or agreeably, to sudden changes in habit. When nature starts to 'clean house' the person concerned generally feels worse for several days. Unfortunately, this feeling is generally interpreted to mean that the treatment is wrong — that it is doing more harm than good. This is quite a mistaken idea. You know what a home is like during the process of spring cleaning. It is in a state of chaos. But when the job is finished and everything is restored to its right place, the house looks wonderfully neat and clean.

So it is with the body. The dietetic changes recommended by nutritional science are comparable to a spring cleaning. We are invariably upset by it. But if we persevere, an abiding sense of well-being takes possession of us in due course, and finally we get well. And once restored to health, it is easy, armed with the new knowledge of nutritional science, to stay well.

The Healing Crisis

As the sufferer's blood pressure increases, his mental qualities often become dulled so that he is seldom fully aware of all his disabilities. This is one of the difficulties in obtaining his co-operation in remedial measures. He may not realize the full extent or seriousness of his illness.

As his health is slowly restored, his mental faculties become more acute and he notices areas of pain and discomfort which had previously not troubled him, or had bothered him only slightly.

During the period of transition from sickness to health there is thus a phase that may really be unpleasant. Pains that had not been felt by the sufferer for years, will probably reassert themselves. These pains actually mark a retracting of the steps towards health and although the recurrence of sundry pains is generally a symptom of improving health, this phase rarely evokes any enthusiasm from the sufferer. It is during this period that those helping the sufferer find their experience and resources are taxed to the utmost to convince him to continue with the remedial measures outlined in this book.

The Rice Diet 'Cure'

From drugs and surgery, an orthodox craze for the alleged 'cure' of high blood pressure is the rice diet.

The patient is obliged to eat nine ounces of rice every day — no meat, no bread, no milk, cheese, fish, salt or vegetables. The only other articles of food and drink allowed are quantities of fruit and fruit juices. Good results have been claimed for this diet and, no doubt, it would produce better results than the usual drug treatment. The fact that protein foods are cut out, and that abundant fruit and fruit juices are insisted upon, would have a most salutary effect in reducing blood pressure.

The chief virtue in the rice, from the point of view of high blood pressure, is that it is a relatively salt-free food.

The weakness of the 'rice diet', of course, is that any good result from it would be of a temporary nature. Its lack of variety, to say nothing of its chemical imbalance, would cause people to tire of it and drift back to the old tradition.

However, the experiment with rice, fruit and fruit juices is a definite advance on the use of drugs.

Professor Edward McCollum, one of the great medical scientists of the famous Johns Hopkins University, had this to say on the subject of high blood pressure: 'Diversion is a cure for all types of worry, fear, anxiety, jealousy and regret. If one finds himself worrying, that is the time to read a book, mop a floor, visit a neighbour, do some shopping, mend an umbrella, clean the fish bowl, bathe the dog. Sometimes small worries are over-exaggerated by over-sensitive nerves. This might indicate calcium starvation. Check up on the calcium supply. See that there is ample calcium in your diet.

'Hardened arteries and subsequent high blood pressure may be aggravated by a partial failure on the part of the organs of the body burdened with the responsibility of eliminating waste or refuse material. The bowels should be kept fully open at all times. The kidneys should be flushed with fresh, clear, cool drinking water, for which there is no substitute. The skin and glands of perspiration must be considered as organs of elimination. The skin should be kept well and frequently cleansed and invigorated by massage and exposure to sun and air.

'A person suffering from high blood pressure or hardened arteries should not engage in the wild gyrations of the average gymnasium, but should, rather, take short walks in the sunshine and engage in complete and free movement of the entire body while walking.

'These walks should never be tiring, but terminated long before the energy is exhausted. Regular hours of exercise, rest and sleep should be developed by the person suffering from high blood pressure, and nothing should be allowed to infringe upon these established habits.

Professor McCollum On Diet

'The diet, until recovery, should largely consist of fresh green, leafy vegetables, sun-ripened fruits and berries in their freshest form. Dairy products such as milk, cream, unsalted butter and cottage cheese are desirable in moderation.

'All nuts (except chestnuts and peanuts) may be taken as a source of protein to prevent a loss of weight. For the same purpose an ample supply of grapes, grape juice, raisins and various types of soya bean foods and drinks should be included in the diet, as these foods aid in body building without the danger of toxic accumulation so frequently accompanying the overuse of meat, fish, eggs, fowl and heavy manufactured cheeses, when the organs of the body are too tired or unable to successfully handle them.

'To sum up the fight against high blood pressure: Quit worrying; bathe frequently; keep the bowels open; exercise mildly in the sunshine; eat abundantly of fruits, vegetables, fruit juices, vegetable juices, nuts, dairy products etc. Diminish the use of fish and flesh foods as well as all foods of a toxic nature. Drink water, develop regular hours of sleep and rest, as well as regular hours for work, and don't get excited about your blood pressure.'

Two Cautions
Of the importance of diet in the cure of high blood pressure, Dr Howard Hay writes: 'Two more cautions are necessary. One is to make sure that you have plenty of vitamins and minerals, so be certain to eat raw food freely, salads, fruits, vegetables, even the grains; if you like, a little oatmeal with nuts or raisins and honey mixed with it.

'The other caution is not to go too far with fats, for while they have nothing to do with the formation of blood pressure, yet the body is not intended to subsist very largely on fats or oils except in the very cold weather, so two ounces of fats or oils a day is about all that you can handle easily.

'Avoid white flour and white sugar and all processed starches, for they rob you of the things you need, and you would starve to death on them in about the same time as if you took nothing at all, as has been many times proved.

'If you are constipated, as you almost surely are, this plan of diet will cure you in time: but do not wait for this time, as your colon is filled with decaying filth, so get busy with the enema, washing out the colon every night before retiring with a full two quarts of cool water, all retained at once, and do this till there is a regular daily stool before the time for enema, when it will not be necessary any longer.

'Now if you have been worrying about blood pressure forget it, for very few cases are too far gone not to get well again, or certainly to hold the condition down and live out life successfully and happily.'

A most important point to remember is this: The body — and all its parts — is constantly renewing itself. Every day two or three ounces of dead tissue cells — the dead tissue of bone, muscle, nerves, arterial walls, and organs — are passed out of the body. And every day these dead tissue cells are being replaced by new cells from the food we eat.

If the food we eat is right — if it has sufficient protein for worn-out tissue replacement, but no more than that; if it contains all the necessary vitamins and organic minerals for pure blood and efficient glandular and organic functioning, then it can be said that the body is slowly rebuilding itself, renewing itself and repairing the damaged parts.

The new connective tissue for the arteries will be of a highly elastic and resilient quality, and a form of 'invisible mending' will take place. By this amazing process, nature builds tissue to heal wounds, rebuilds injured parts, renews defective organs, and knits bones.

It is generally agreed by physiologists that the entire

body is completely renewed every seven years. Therefore to suffering humanity, we say, go ye and eat wisely and re-new yourself!

The Emotional Factors

In the foregoing pages, we have put most of the emphasis upon the physical, i.e., the nutritional aspect of cause and cure. But the emotional or psychological aspects are also important.

If you could examine the wall of a blood vessel under a microscope, you would notice that a network of tiny nerves is an essential part of its structure. Therefore, any emotion — anger, frustration, impatience, etc. — which affects the nerves, causes them to contract or dilate the blood vessels. An outburst of such emotion, affecting the entire nervous organization can quickly raise the blood pressure to danger point. To overcome these emotional upsets we can only suggest two things:

1. An objective attempt to control them.
2. A scheme of life which feeds the starved nerves and relaxes their tension.

No. 2 can be achieved by building up the health in general and by supplying the B-complex vitamins and calcium.

However, no. 1 is more difficult. It demands that the person concerned changes his temperament, and that is not easy. Only he can make the attempt.

Summary of Corrective Principles

Let us take all the corrective principles set out in this book:

1. Reduce protein food (meat, eggs, fish and cheese) to not more than three to four ounces daily.

2. Reduce all animal fats to the minimum.

3. Eat less and eat simply, thus giving the circulatory system the smallest possible task compatible with your minimum food requirements.

4. Greatly reduce or cut out altogether the clogging starchy foods, such as white bread, processed breakfast foods, biscuits, cake, etc.

5. Cut out all tinned foods, sausage meats, hamburgers, pies, pastries, corned beef, recooked foods, lollies, etc.

6. Cut out all condiments — mustard, Worcester sauce, salt and pepper, etc.

7. Cut out alcohol, tea, coffee, cocoa. When you are feeling better, a cup of weak tea twice daily will not hurt. Meanwhile, drink freely of diluted orange and lemon juice, or raw vegetable juices. No sugar.

8. Eat no fried foods.

9. Make the 80-20 formula your basic principle of diet. That is to say, see that your diet consists of approximately 80 per cent of alkaline-forming foods (fruit, salads, vegetables and dried fruits) and only about 20 per cent of acid-forming foods (meat, eggs, cheese, fish, breadstuffs and cereals).

10. The foregoing diet is rich in alkalines and vitamins. A blood stream rich in these two magic substances will gradually dissolve the deposits of cholesterol and urate salts on the arterial walls, as well as the fibrosis, and allow the blood to circulate more freely.

11. A diet rich in vitamins and minerals also ensures that the glands and organs of the body function efficiently, thus assisting digestion, stimulating the nervous system, the peristaltic action of the intestines, and eliminating waste matter.

12. Regular elimination is essential — without the aid of pills or purgatives. The diet suggested in this book will do this (with the help of molasses, if necessary) after the meal.

13. Give yourself a good brisk tone up with a skin brush after your bath each day.

14. Smoking and alcohol should either be cut out altogether, or reduced to a mere gesture.

15. Finally, vitamin E is essential to the restoration of normal functioning of the circulatory mechanism, and vitamins B_1, B-complex, C, vitamin A and D capsules, calcium (white) tablets, kelp tablets, and lecithin capsules are important aids to recovery.

For the rest, the recovery of the blood pressure sufferer is chiefly psychological. He must take things easier and cultivate relaxation — particularly in the open air. He must learn not to take himself quite so seriously. He must cultivate a cheerful disposition and not worry. He simply cannot afford to allow little matters — or big ones — to upset or anger him.

Armed with this mental attitude, and with the principles set out in this book, any sufferer from high blood pressure can usually recover by consistently applying these principles and making them part of his daily life for the next twelve months.

He will find such improvement that he will never go back to the old way of eating and living. He will be on the road to permanent recovery.

One final word of warning: There is no other known road to recovery. Other methods have failed to permanently remove the cause of high blood pressure.

Specific Diets to Help Control Hypertension

i. *Low-salt Diet*

The first consideration must be to decrease the amount of sodium (i.e. salt) intake yet maintain an adequate energy intake. This diet will provide 60 to 90g of protein (1,000-2,000 calories), yet the sodium intake is only that necessary for health.

Sample Daily Menu

Breakfast: Fruit or fruit juice, unsweetened
Low-salt cereal or muesli
Milk and sugar from allowance
One egg (unsalted)
Low-sodium bread as toast
Low-salt butter or soft margarine from allowance
Preserve or marmalade or honey
Weak tea or decaffeinated coffee with milk from allowance and preferably unsweetened

Midday meal: Fruit or fruit juice, unsweetened
3 oz (75g) unsalted meat, poultry or white fish, grilled or fried in vegetable oils
Potato or rice or pasta
Fresh or frozen vegetables, boiled without added salt
Salad with vegetable oil dressing
Low-sodium bread with butter or soft margarine from allowance
Fruit with honey
Weak tea with milk from allowance and preferably unsweetened

Evening meal: Fruit or fruit juice
2 oz (60g) unsalted meat or fish
Fresh or frozen vegetables or salad
Low-sodium bread or roll with butter or
    soft margarine from allowance
Weak tea with milk from allowance and
    preferably unsweetened
Bedtime: Remainder of milk allowance
Allowance Milk — ½ pint (250ml)
for day: Butter or soft magarine — 1 oz (30g)
    with low-salt content.

General Considerations

No salt to be used in cooking or at table. Avoid all cured meat and fish e.g. bacon, ham, tongue, pickled brisket and silverside; smoked fish of any kind, tinned fish; all canned meats, vegetables and soups; cheeses, bottled sauces, pickles, sausages; all foods made with bicarbonate of soda or baking powder such as cakes and biscuits; seasoning salts and sea salt.

All labels of processed foods should be checked and must be avoided if they contain salt (including sea salt), sodium bicarbonate, sodium benzoate and monosodium glutamate. Use of low-sodium milk will decrease the intake of sodium.

The diet gives a good intake of potassium which helps nullify the effect of previous high sodium levels. If the individual finds the diet unappetizing, it is possible to use salt-substitutes which contain potassium chloride.

Further energy requirements are best met with extra honey. Raw sugar should be used as a sweetener with absence of honey.

ii. *Diet to Lower Blood Cholesterol*

The basis of this diet is a reduction in the intake of saturated fats and cholesterol and an increase in poly-unsaturated oils. It is adequate in all nutrients with the exception of iron. This is best taken in supplementary form as Iron Amino Acid Chelate (one tablet with each meal).

Sample Daily Menu

Breakfast: Fruit or fruit juice, unsweetened

Muesli or cereal or porridge with skimmed milk and honey (if sweetener is required)

Toast

Soft poly-unsaturated margarine and preserve or honey

Weak tea or decaffeinated coffee with skimmed milk and raw sugar (if required)

Mid-morning: Weak tea or decaffeinated coffee with skimmed milk and raw sugar (if required)

Mid-afternoon: Fruit or fruit juice, unsweetened

Evening meal: Poultry, fish or lean meat cooked in poly-unsaturated vegetable oil

Potatoes or rice or pasta

Vegetables, raw or cooked or salad

Bread or plain roll with poly-unsaturated margarine

Fruit or dessert (any that are milk-free with no animal fat)

Decaffeinated coffee or weak tea with skimmed milk and raw sugar

Bedtime: Skimmed milk or fruit juice
                  Crackers with a little peanut butter

General Considerations

Foods to be avoided: Butter and hard margarines, lard, suet and shortenings and all cakes, biscuits and pastry made with these; fatty meat, meat pies, sausages and luncheon meats; whole milk and cream, commercial cream toppings, chocolate and ice-cream; cheese with the exception of low-fat cottage cheese, coconut, coconut oil and coffee whiteners; organ meats such as liver, kidneys and brain; fish roe, caviar and shrimp; foods fried in animal fats. Eat no more than two eggs per week.

Foods allowed: Wholemeal bread, crispbreads and plain biscuits; breakfast cereals, muesli, porridge; pasta, potatoes and rice; all vegetables and pulses, salads and fruit; fish, baked or fried in poly-unsaturated oil; lean meat, preferably veal, chicken or turkey; all preserves and honey; tea, decaffeinated coffee and fruit drinks; all poly-unsaturated oils and margarines; skimmed milk and low-fat yogurt; cottage cheese and skimmed milk cheese; meringues, cakes and biscuits made with egg white, skimmed milk and poly-unsaturated oils.

Beef, lamb, ham and pork should be limited to three helpings (each of 3 oz or 90g) per week and all visible fat must be removed.

For baking, use only poly-unsaturated oils and fats. Egg whites and skimmed milk must be used.

Final Word

The high blood pressure sufferer, if he is wise, will slow down the tempo of his life. He will take things easier. He will cultivate a more equable and philosophical attitude.

He will cultivate the art of relaxing. He is counselled to apply the principles set out in this book intelligently and consistently, but not to become a slave to them. If he does the right thing nine times out of ten, nature will forgive the odd fall from grace.

Let us end on this very positive note: the principles laid down in this book represent the proved and approved principles of modern nutritional science. They fail only in that small percentage of cases which are too far gone to recover. If you are not in this bracket, then you have every reason and every right to expect improvement; but you must be patient and consistent. A small improvement can be effected quickly, but this condition can only be corrected over a long period of time.

This book has told you what modern science knows. High blood pressure can be overcome and *is* being overcome. It is now up to you.

Index